Rejuvenate Your Body: Lose Weight and Heal with a Carnivore Diet."

Amanda B. Coats

INTRODUCTION

Juliet, a youthful lady on an adventure for a superior life, lived in the center of an active city where the scent of distinctive sorts of nourishment blended together.

With everything going off-base in her life right presently, she finished up needing changes, not a short-term objective.
 There was a point when, while perusing a parcel of food-related articles and books, she came across a progressive thought: the Carnivore Eat less.

 She got to be interested in this arbitrary way of eating and learned that it may offer assistance in losing weight as well as recuperate her and make her cheerful in common.

This book is not fair and direct to cooking; it's too a travel into the universes of wellbeing and basics. In this authentic book, we welcome you to connect us on an investigation of the chasing way of life.

You will learn how to utilize the control of animal-based nourishment to your claim advantage.

Envision having perpetual vitality, a sound intellect, and a body that feels light and speedy when you wake up each day. Envision brilliant dinners that not as it were taste extraordinary but too offer assistance from the interior out.

This book is your ticket to this recently found need. It's a treasure trove of scrumptious formulas and carefully arranged suppers that are implied to offer assistance when you reach your weight misfortune objectives, move forward your generally wellbeing, and speed up recuperating from the interior out. There is a wide run of formulas in this book, from top notch steaks to top notch angle suppers. All of them are outlined to fit the prerequisites of the Meat Eater Count calories.

Each formula is carefully organized to entice your sense of taste as well as outfit your body with the essential supplements it needs. From liberal morning dinners to satisfying dinners, our formulas are an occasion of the flood and extravagance that the set of all creatures brings to the table. However, this book is something other than a grouping of formulas.

A helper empowers you to accept command over your prosperity and riches. We share the science behind the Carnivore Count calories, loosening up the fantasies and perplexities that encompass it.

You'll discover how this count of calories can be a necessary resource for weight decrease, tending to continuous therapeutic issues, and progressing recovering in ways you never envisioned.

As you take off on this groundbreaking outing, we empower you to grasp the Meat eater count calories not as a basic culinary choice, but or maybe as a total way of life alteration

It's a request to reconnect with the ordinary, fundamental faculties that exist in us all - inclinations that direct us toward perfect prosperity and essentialness. By and by, as you get a handle on this book, we encourage you to move out toward a way better, more happy you.

Grasp this book with an open heart and a curious intellect. Let the formulas inside these pages be your driving light, edifying the way toward a day by day presence stacked up with wellbeing and flood. Is it safe to say that you are arranged to take off on this modern trip?

The capacity to alter your life is inside your hands. Turn the page, hop into the universe of the book - Rejuvenate Your Body: Lose Weight and Heal with a Carnivore Diet, and let the travel begin. Your body, intellect, and soul will thank you for it.

Click, add to cart and purchase your copy to start reaping the benefits NOW.

CHAPTER 1

What is the Diet Of Carnivores?

The strict carnivore diet consists only of meat, fish, eggs, and some dairy products. All other foods, fruits, vegetables, grains, legumes, nuts, and seeds are banned.

Lawyers of this approach Also recommend limiting or barring dairy input to lactose-free foods like hard rubbish and adulation.

The carnivore diet is grounded on the contentious proposition that high- carb diets are to   be condemned for the high   frequency of habitual sickness in the moment and that meat and fish were the main foods consumed by the ancient societies.

Some well- known low- carb rules, like the paleo and ketogenic diets,   circumscribe but don't fully exclude carb input, still, the thing of the carnivorous diet is to avoid carbs.

How precisely does the diet of herbivores operate?

This kind of ketogenic diet consists solely of eating meat, fish, eggs, and small quantities of low- lactose dairy products. It Also excludes all plant- produced foods.

Respectable   effects include funk, bomb, overindulge,   angel,   meat,   organ   meat, oleaginous and white fish, hard scrap, adoration, and milk.

Adipose slices of beef are advised by attorneys to   satisfy   quotidian   energy   conditions. Typically, our bodies produce energy using glucose, which comes from carbohydrate sources.

A state known as ketosis arises when there's inadequate glucose. In this script, lipids replace carbohydrates as the body's main energy source. Analogous to a carnivorous diet, when we hesitate from carbohydrates, the liver converts fat stores into" ketones," which are our body's source of energy.

The carnivore diet encourages blood sugar regulation, weight loss, and better mood. It was erected on the premise that diets high in carbohydrates are the main contributor to habitual illness. Still, eating nothing but animal protein and no carbohydrates has downsides.

Carbs take on an awful personality. Your body turns carbs into glucose, which it needs as energy, throughout digestion. Still, those carbs will snappily turn into fat if you do not exercise regularly. Thus, consuming an   inordinate quantum of carbs may result in weight gain."

Carbohydrates are your body's favored energy source what it's acquainted to using for energy," the nations of Patton." Still, burning fat is your coming stylish volition if you avoid eating carbohydrates. And this happens whether you burn fat from your own body fat or from the meals you eat.

According to her, people feel more when they cut out on carbohydrates because eating meat is less   inflammatory and their blood sugar situations do not change as much. Still, she cautions that ingesting an inordinate quantity of animal fat may Also beget inflammation.

Not every carbohydrate is dangerous or equal. When they're at their utmost introductory, carbohydrates give your body energy. Multitudinous nutritional carbohydrates that are rich in fiber, vitamins, and minerals are Also available.

The stylish carbs are those that are neither repurposed or perfected, and are closest to their natural state.

Suppose many of the following apples, pineapples, and strawberries are exemplifications of fruits. Carrots, sweet potatoes, and beets are exemplifications of vegetables. Complete grains, similar to whole wheat chuck and quinoa.

Steer clear of simple carbs like those set up in pies, galettes, sweet treats, and sticky treats. These are known to beget inflammation and weight gain, especially around the midriff, and are frequently heavy in white sugar, wheat, and preservatives. Also, obesity, high blood pressure, and Type 2 diabetes — which results in oscillations in blood sugar have all been linked to these carbs.

Naturally, barring them from your diet can make you feel more because you will exfoliate pounds and experience less oscillations in blood sugar situations. Still, for health reasons, you do not have to hesitate from all carbohydrates. In actuality, you could seriously harm your health by doing so.

What pitfalls come with eating a carnivorous diet?

There's some description of the carnivorous diet. Also, there will be serious impacts if you count entire food groups from your diet." The carnivore diet is super low in fiber, which will beget a lot of constipation," Patton stated. And the impacts escalate beyond simply forgetting to urinate. Complications, similar as elevated blood pressure and cholesterol," If you have apre- being habitual condition." In fact, the high protein and fat content of this diet, which takes longer to digest, may complicate digestive problems."

Why Did You Choose This Diet?

There are some who have set up success with a carnivorous diet. While some people have only used it compactly, others have used it sometimes.

Since there's a lack of significant scientific exploration on the flesh-only diet, we must calculate people's descriptions in order to better understand why they stick to it.

Thankfully, the reports are attainable, and they are appealing. Individuals witness rapid-fire weight loss, bettered digestion, internal clarity, and indeed the resolution of some autoimmune conditions.

But flash back that numerous of these people didn't start out eating carnivorously; rather, it was a last resort.

Let's examine more closely at how this diet might give similar advantages. You can lose weight by following a carnivorous diet. Current exploration indicates that meals high in protein are relatively salutary in both precluding and saying hunger. Eating a large portion of red meat is one of the stylish ways to gain a lot of high-quality protein. Suppose that is what you eat for every meal during the day.

Eating meat causes you to feel fuller faster and consume less calories because it keeps your brain from receiving negative signals when you eat the same meal again and over.

Initial accounts from the carnivorous community corroborate this reasoning. Adherents of the carnivorous diet tend to be less hungry and report having smaller waistlines.

Additionally, people usually mention eating fewer meals a day—usually two or perhaps just one—consistently. People who do this are able to develop a sweet deficit, which is essential for losing weight and eventually reducing body fat.

It can aid in the treatment of autoimmune diseases. There are other beneficial aspects of having a sweet deficit as well. It decreases blood sugar levels, enhances insulin sensitivity, and increases autophagy, the body's process of eliminating metabolic waste. This thus lowers inflammation and often relieves the symptoms associated with autoimmune complaints.

Research also demonstrates that in only two days, including meat into your diet and adopting a carnivorous diet can dramatically change your gut's beneficial bacterial population, known as the gut microbiota. While research on the connection between bacteria and human health is still in its early stages, it has already revealed that a healthy microbiota is associated with a decreased risk of having habitual seditious disorders.

Additionally, there may be defenses against autoimmunity. It is gentle on the digestive system. For the majority of people, having a healthy digestive system is correlated with consuming adequate beneficial fiber.

Unfortunately, eating a lot of stringy foods like veggies can sometimes make individuals with major digestive problems—such as a seditious bowel complaint (IBD) or twisted bowel pattern (IBS)—feel worse.

If one's stomach was previously inflamed, it might still be mechanically bruised by fiber, which is why persons with these disorders are often advised to follow a low-residue diet. The majority of residue, which passes through the whole digestive system undigested, is made up of fiber. The carnivore diet is the best low-residue diet since it has little fiber and is ideal for people with comparable issues.

The carnivorous diet is beneficial for brain function. Adipose cuts of meat are typically preferred by those following a carnivorous diet since they contain no carbs and may be used as a primary source of fat energy. This increases their likelihood of entering ketosis, along with the fact that they often only eat once or twice a day. When the body doesn't obtain enough carbs from the food, it transitions to burning fat instead of carbohydrates, which is known as nutritional ketosis.

Carnivore diets may have similar advantages as ketogenic diets, since they have been demonstrated to aid with diabetes and many neurological   illnesses.

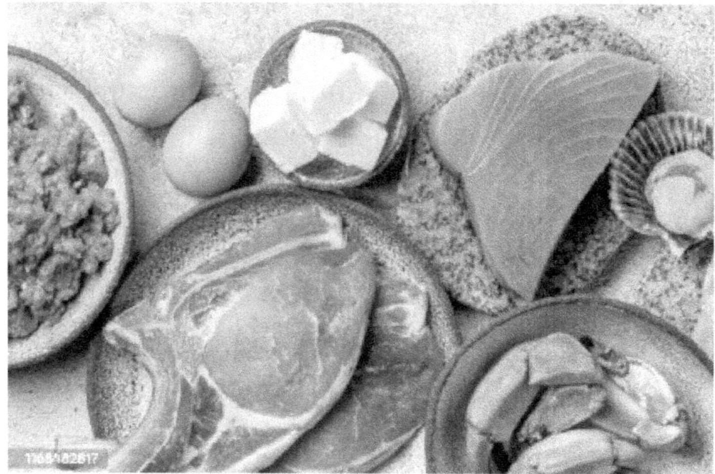

CHAPTER 2

Principles of Eating Carnivorously

The carnivorous diet, often referred to as a zero-carb or all-meat diet, is a healthful strategy that forbids meals made in factories and promotes the use of animal products. It is based on the idea that humans originated as herbivores, or at the very least, as animal-like creatures that consumed a lot of animal food. The carnivorous diet's proponents contend that it may result in a variety of vibrant health advantages, including decreased inflammation, improved internal clarity, and weight loss.

The Foundations of an Insatiable Diet

(1) **Emphasis on Foods Derived from Animals**: Eating mostly animal-based foods, such as meat, fish, eggs, and certain dairy products like trash and milk, is the cornerstone of a carnivorous diet. These foods are abundant in the vital lipids, vitamins, minerals, and protein needed for good health.

(2) **Foods derived from plants only:** In contrast to other health-promoting strategies that incorporate an assortment of fruits, vegetables, grains, and legumes, the carnivorous diet eliminates all processed foods. Fruits, vegetables, grains, legumes, nuts, seeds, and canvases that have been inferred from stores are included in this.

(3) **Highlight Viscosity of nutrients:** It's critical to give nutrient-dense animal foods first priority while eating a carnivorous diet. In conclusion, look for premium meats like organ meat, pasturage-raised beef, wild-caught fish, and lawn-fed beef. Numerous vital elements, such as protein, iron, zinc, vitamin B12, and omega-3 adipose acids, are provided by these meals.

(4) **Pay Attention to Your Body:** A fundamental tenet of the carnivorous diet is to pay attention to your body's indications of malnourishment and hunger. Many people discover that eating a carnivorous diet naturally makes them feel less hungry all the time and results in smaller jones since animal foods are generally filling. Observe your reactions to various meals and adjust your diet accordingly.

(5) **Be Hydrated:** A carnivorous diet requires you to be sufficiently hydrated, even if meat includes some water. To sustain adequate hydration conditions and promote general health and well-being, sip water throughout the day.

(6) **Take Supplements:** Even while animal foods offer a wide range of nutrients, certain individuals may benefit from taking supplements when following a carnivorous diet. Electrolytes, magnesium, potassium, and vitamin D are important nutrients to take into account. See a medical practitioner to find out whether you need any supplements based on your specific needs.

(7) **Examine instances involving electrolytes**: Because a carnivorous diet removes many of the electrolyte sources that are often present in factory-ground meals, it's critical to monitor your electrolyte levels and ensure appropriate intake. It is especially crucial to focus on the electrolytes sodium, potassium, and magnesium if you have symptoms like headaches, exhaustion, or cramping in your muscles.

(8) **Practice Proper Food Preparation:** Proper food preparation is essential when following a carnivorous diet to ensure food safety and maximize nutrient absorption. Cook meat thoroughly to eliminate harmful bacteria and pathogens, and opt for cooking methods such as grilling, roasting, or slow cooking to enhance flavor and texture.

(9) **Be Mindful of Food Quality:** Quality matters when it comes to the carnivorous diet. Opt for high-quality, organic, grass-fed, pasture-raised, and wild-caught animal products whenever possible. These foods tend to be more nutrient-dense and free from antibiotics, hormones, and other harmful additives.

(10)**Stay Flexible:** While the carnivorous diet primarily focuses on animal-based foods, it's essential to stay flexible and listen to your body's needs. Some individuals may find that they thrive on a strict carnivorous diet, while others may benefit from occasional deviations or additions such as bone broth, fermented dairy, or small amounts of plant-based foods.

The carnivorous diet is a dietary approach that emphasizes the consumption of animal-based foods while excluding plant-based foods. By focusing on nutrient-dense animal products, listening to your body's hunger and satiety signals, and practicing proper food preparation, you can enjoy the potential health benefits of a carnivorous diet. However, it's essential to stay flexible and consult with a healthcare professional to ensure that the carnivorous diet is appropriate for your individual needs and health goals.

Ways to get ready for a carnivorous diet.

Embarking on a carnivorous diet requires careful preparation and consideration to ensure a smooth transition and optimal health outcomes. Whether you're new to the concept or transitioning from a different dietary approach, taking proactive steps to prepare for the carnivorous diet can help set you up for success.

Before diving into the carnivorous diet, it's essential to understand its principles and potential benefits. Research the science behind the diet, including its historical context, nutritional composition, and potential health implications. Familiarize yourself with the foods allowed on the carnivorous diet, such as meat, fish, eggs, and certain dairy products, as well as foods to avoid, including fruits, vegetables, grains, legumes, nuts, seeds, and plant-derived oils.

Consult with a Healthcare Professional.

Before making any significant dietary changes, consult with a healthcare professional, such as a doctor, nutritionist, or dietitian. They can provide personalized guidance based on your medical history, current health status, and individual nutritional needs. Discuss your intentions to adopt a carnivorous diet and address any potential concerns or considerations, such as nutrient deficiencies, food allergies, or underlying health conditions.

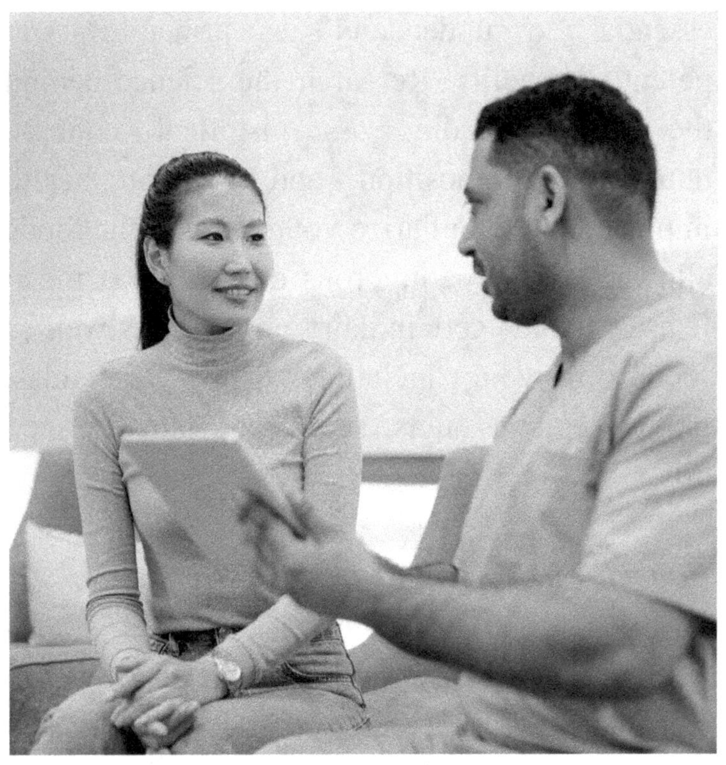

Gradual Transition.

Transitioning to a carnivorous diet can be a significant adjustment for your body, both physically and mentally. Consider easing into the diet gradually rather than making abrupt changes overnight.

Start by gradually reducing the consumption of plant-based foods while increasing your intake of animal-based foods. This gradual transition can help minimize potential digestive discomfort and withdrawal symptoms associated with eliminating carbohydrates and plant foods from your diet.

Educate Yourself on Nutrient Needs.

Animal-based foods provide a rich array of essential nutrients necessary for optimal health, including protein, vitamins, minerals, and healthy fats. Educate yourself on the nutrient composition of different animal foods and how they contribute to your overall nutritional needs.

Pay particular attention to nutrients that may be lacking in a carnivorous diet, such as fiber, vitamin C, potassium, and certain antioxidants. Explore alternative sources or supplementation strategies to ensure you're meeting your nutritional requirements.

Plan Your Meals

Meal planning is crucial for success on a carnivorous diet. Take the time to plan your meals and snacks in advance, ensuring they're balanced, satisfying, and aligned with your dietary goals. Incorporate a variety of animal-based foods, including different types of meat, fish, poultry, and eggs, to ensure a diverse nutrient intake. Experiment with different cooking methods, seasonings, and recipes to keep your meals interesting and enjoyable.

Stock Up on Essentials

Prepare your kitchen and pantry by stocking up on essential ingredients for a carnivorous diet.

Invest in high-quality animal products, including grass-fed beef, pasture-raised poultry, wild-caught fish, organ meats, and quality eggs. Consider purchasing in bulk or sourcing from local farmers or specialty suppliers for the freshest and most nutrient-dense options. Additionally, stock up on cooking fats such as tallow, lard, butter, and ghee for cooking and flavoring your meals.

Stay Hydrated

Hydration is key to overall health and well-being, especially when following a carnivorous diet. While animal-based foods contain some water, it's essential to drink plenty of fluids throughout the day to maintain optimal hydration levels. Choose water as your primary beverage and avoid sugary drinks, caffeinated beverages, and artificial additives. Consider adding electrolytes or mineral-rich salts to your water to support hydration and replenish essential nutrients lost through sweating and urination.

Prepare for Detoxification Symptoms

As your body adjusts to the carnivorous diet and eliminates toxins and metabolic waste accumulated from previous dietary habits, you may experience detoxification symptoms such as fatigue, headaches, irritability, or digestive disturbances. Be prepared for these temporary discomforts and take steps to support your body's natural detoxification processes. Get plenty of rest, stay hydrated, practice stress-reducing activities like meditation or gentle exercise, and consider incorporating detoxifying practices such as sauna sessions or dry brushing.

Monitor Your Progress

Keep track of your progress and how you're feeling physically, mentally, and emotionally as you transition to a carnivorous diet. Monitor changes in your energy levels, mood, digestion, sleep quality, and overall well-being. Keep a food diary to record your meals, portion sizes, and any symptoms or reactions you experience. Adjust your dietary approach as needed based on your observations and consult with a healthcare professional if you have any concerns or questions.

Seek Support and Community

Joining a supportive community of like-minded individuals can provide encouragement, motivation, and valuable resources as you navigate the carnivorous diet. Seek out online forums, social media groups, or local meetups dedicated to carnivorous eating where you can share experiences, ask questions, and learn from others on similar journeys. Having a supportive network can make the transition to a carnivorous diet feel less daunting and more sustainable in the long run.

CHAPTER 3

What to Eat

When considering a carnivorous diet, it's essential to understand the principles behind it and how to optimize your nutrition within its confines.

A carnivorous diet, also known as a zero carb or all-meat diet, primarily consists of animal products such as meat, fish, and eggs, while excluding plant-based foods. While this may seem restrictive, there's a surprising variety of foods to choose from within these categories.

- **MEAT**

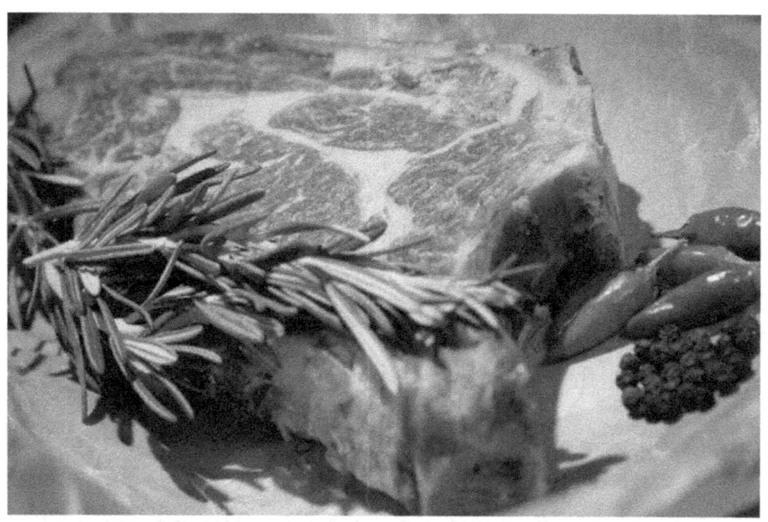

Types of Meat
1. **Beef**
 Beef is a staple of the carnivore diet due to its high fat and protein content. Opt for fatty cuts like ribeye, chuck roast, or brisket for maximum satiety and nutrient density.

2. **Pork**

Pork provides a delicious alternative to beef, with options such as bacon, pork chops, and pork belly. Like beef, choose fattier cuts to maintain energy levels and promote ketosis.

3. **Poultry**

Chicken and turkey are leaner options, making them suitable for those looking to control fat intake. Thighs and wings are higher in fat compared to breast meat, making them preferable choices on a carnivorous diet.

4. **Lamb**

Lamb offers a unique flavor profile and is rich in essential nutrients like zinc and vitamin B12. Lamb chops, shoulder, and leg are excellent choices for carnivores.

5. **Game Meat**

Venison, bison, and elk are leaner options packed with protein and essential vitamins and minerals. While less common, they provide variety and can be a delicious addition to a carnivorous diet.

6. **Organ Meats**

Liver, heart, kidney, and other organ meats are nutritional powerhouses, providing essential vitamins and minerals like vitamin A, B vitamins, iron, and zinc. Incorporating these into your diet ensures you're getting a broad spectrum of nutrients.

- **FISH AND SEAFOOD**

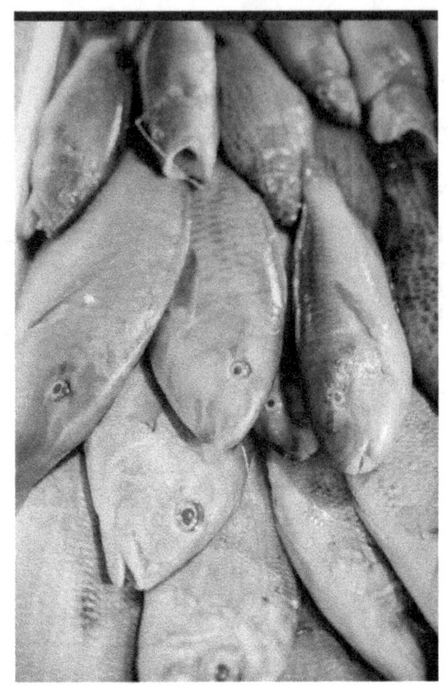

1. **Salmon**

Rich in omega-3 fatty acids, salmon is an excellent choice for cardiovascular health and overall well-being. Opt for wild-caught salmon whenever possible to minimize exposure to contaminants.

2. **Sardines**

These small fish are packed with nutrients like omega-3s, calcium, and vitamin D. Canned sardines are convenient and budget-friendly, making them a practical choice for carnivores.

3. **Mackerel**

Another fatty fish high in omega-3s, mackerel provides a flavorful addition to a carnivorous diet. Enjoy it grilled, baked, or pan-fried for a delicious and nutritious meal.

4. **Shrimp**

Shrimp are low in calories and carbohydrates while being rich in protein and essential nutrients like selenium and iodine. They're quick to cook and versatile, making them an excellent option for carnivores.

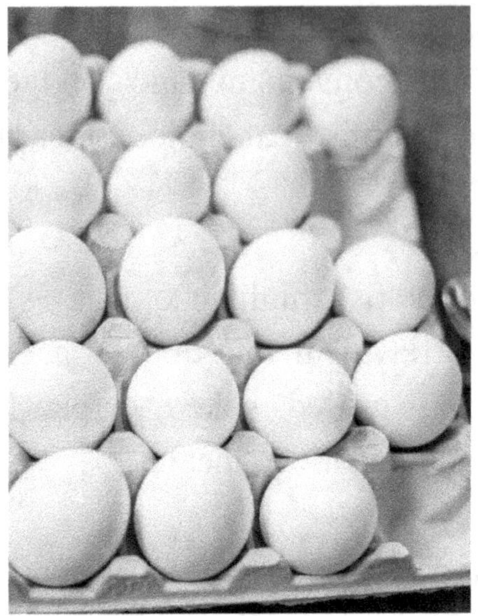

1. **Chicken Eggs:** Eggs are a complete protein source and versatile ingredient that can be enjoyed in various ways, including boiled, fried, scrambled, or as part of omelets and frittatas.

2. **Duck Eggs:** Duck eggs offer a larger yolk and richer flavor compared to chicken eggs. They're an excellent alternative for those looking to switch things up in their carnivorous diet.

3. **Quail Eggs:** Quail eggs are smaller in size but pack a nutritional punch with high levels of protein, vitamins, and minerals. They can be enjoyed boiled, fried, or pickled as a tasty snack or appetizer.

- **FATS**

1. **Tallow**: Tallow is rendered beef fat that can be used for cooking or as a flavorful addition to dishes. It's high in saturated fats and provides a rich, savory flavor to meats and vegetables.

2. **Lard**: Similar to tallow, lard is rendered pork fat commonly used in cooking and baking. It adds moisture and flavor to dishes and is a staple in many traditional cuisines.

3. **Butter and Ghee**: Butter and ghee (clarified butter) are rich in fat-soluble vitamins like A, D, E, and K2. They add richness and depth to dishes and can be used for frying, sautéing, or as a topping.

1. **Salt:** Salt is essential for maintaining electrolyte balance on a carnivorous diet, especially during the initial adaptation phase. Opt for high-quality sea salt or Himalayan pink salt to ensure you're getting trace minerals along with sodium.

2. **Black Pepper:** While technically a plant product, black pepper is widely accepted on carnivorous diets due to its minimal impact on overall carb intake. It adds flavor and depth to meats without compromising the principles of the diet.

3. **Bone Broth:** Made by simmering animal bones and connective tissue, bone broth is rich in collagen, gelatin, and minerals like calcium, magnesium, and phosphorus. It's a comforting and nourishing addition to a carnivorous diet, especially during colder months.

- **BEVERAGES**

1. **Water**: Staying hydrated is crucial on a carnivorous diet, so drink plenty of water throughout the day. Opt for filtered or spring water whenever possible to avoid contaminants.

2. **Coffee:** Coffee is generally acceptable on a carnivore diet, though some individuals may prefer to limit or avoid it due to personal preferences or sensitivities. Enjoy it black or with a splash of heavy cream for added richness.

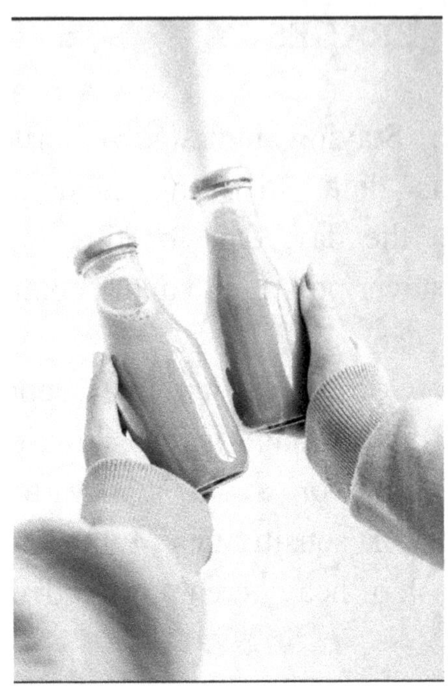

3. **Bone Broth:** In addition to being a food, bone broth can Also be consumed as a beverage, providing hydration along with essential nutrients and electrolytes.

- **SNACKS**

1. **Jerky**: Beef jerky is an accessible and movable snack option that is high in protein and low in carbohydrates. Look for brands without added sugars or artificial constituents for the cleanest option.

2. **Pork Rinds:** Pork rinds are brickle, savory snacks made from fried gormandizer skin. They are carb-free and satisfying, making them an ideal choice for herbivores looking for a brickle treat.

A carnivorous diet offers a different array of foods to enjoy while clinging to its principles of animal - grounded nutrition. By opting for high-quality flesh, fish, eggs, and fats, along with scrumptious seasonings and potables, you can produce satisfying and nutritional meals that support your health and well- being on a carnivorous diet.

As always, listen to your body and acclimate your diet grounded on your individual requirements and preferences.

Opting For Organ Flesh, Fats, and Quality in Animal Proteins

When opting organ flesh, look for fresh, vibrant colors and firm textures. For fats, conclude for sources like avocado, olive oil painting, and adipose fish for healthy options. Quality in animal proteins is pivotal; choose lawn- fed beef, free- range flesh, and wild- caught fish whenever possible for optimal nutrition.

CHAPTER 4

Plan Your Meals and Recipes

Planning your meals and recipes within a carnivorous diet can be both simple and different. While it may feel limited compared to other salutary approaches, a carnivorous diet offers a wide array of options to explore, from colorful cuts of meat to different cuisine styles. This is a detailed companion to help you plan your meals and recipes effectively within a carnivorous frame.

Crucial Nutrients to Consider

When planning meals within a carnivorous diet, it's essential to ensure you are getting a variety of nutrients to support overall health. While animal products are rich in protein and essential fats, they may warrant certain vitamins and minerals generally set up in factory foods.

Tips

1. *Include a variety of meats*

Rotate between different types of animal products to insure you are getting a different range of nutrients. Trial with beef, flesh, seafood, and eggs to keep meals instigative.

2. *Incorporate organ flesh*

Organ flesh are nutrient bootstrappers, rich in vitamins, minerals, and essential nutrients like iron and B vitamins. Include liver, heart, and order in your diet to reap their benefits.

3. *Trial with cuisine styles*

Explore colorful cuisine ways similar as grilling, riding, embroiling, and slow cuisine to enhance flavors and textures. Do not be hysterical to try new fashions and trial with seasonings and gravies.

4. *Prioritize quality*

Whenever possible, choose high- quality, pasturage- raised, and lawn- fed animal products. Not only do they tend to be further nutrient- thick, but they Also support ethical and sustainable husbandry practices.

5. *Listen to your body*

Pay attention to how different foods make you feel and acclimate your diet consequently. While some herbivores thrive on a strict meat-only approach, others may profit from including small quantities of dairy or other animal - deduced foods.

Sample Menus; Simple Herbivore fashions

Then are some simple yet succulent mess ideas to inspire your carnivorous menu planning.

 - *Steak and Eggs*

Start your day with a classic combination of steak and eggs cooked to your relish. Brace a juicy steak with fried or climbed eggs for a satisfying breakfast.

- Grilled Chicken Caesar Salad

Enjoy a stimulating salad featuring grilled funk bone, crisp romaine lettuce, and delicate Caesar dressing. Add grated Parmesan   rubbish for redundant flavor.

- Salmon with Garlic Butter

 Indulge in a   scrumptious regale of grilled or ignited salmon filets   outgunned with garlic adulation   sauce.   Serve   alongside   fumed asparagus or broccoli for a nutritional mess.

- Beef Stir- Fry

 Stir- fry thinly sliced beef with various bell peppers, onions, and mushrooms for a quick and scrumptious   regale. Season with soy sauce, garlic, and gusto for a redundant kick of flavor.

- Bunless Cheeseburgers

 Skip the bun and enjoy juicy cheeseburgers outgunned with your favorite condiments like bacon, avocado, and caramelized onions. Serve with a side of crisp bacon for added crunch.

Planning meals and recipes within a carnivorous diet offers plenty of openings for creativity, variety, and satisfaction. By fasting on nutrient- thick animal products, experimenting with different cuts and cuisine styles, and paying close attention to your body's cues, you can enjoy succulent and nutritional meals while following a rapacious life.

Flash back to prioritize quality, balance, and enjoyment in your salutary choices, and consult with a healthcare professional or nutritionist if you have any specific health enterprises or salutary restrictions.

CHAPTER 5

Difficulties and Resolutions

Embarking on a carnivorous diet can present both challenges and openings for those seeking to borrow this salutary life. While some persons may witness advanced health and well- being, others may encounter difficulties along the way.

In this essay, we will explore the implicit difficulties faced when transitioning to a carnivorous diet and bandy strategies for prostrating these challenges.
One of the primary difficulties persons may encounter when starting a carnivorous diet is the societal perception of similar salutary choices. In a world where factory- grounded diets are frequently promoted as the healthiest option, espousing a diet centered around animal products can be met with dubitation or review from friends, family, and indeed healthcare professionals.

This social pressure can make it challenging for persons to cleave to their salutary preferences and may lead to passions of insulation or disaffection. Another handicap that persons may face when transitioning to a carnivorous diet is the perceived lack of variety in food choices.

Unlike factory- grounded diets, which emphasize a wide array of fruits, vegetables, grains, and legumes, a carnivorous diet primarily consists of meat, fish, eggs, and dairy. Some persons may struggle with humdrum or tedium when eating the same types of foods day after day, leading to jones for variety or a desire to return to further different salutary patterns. Also, persons may encounter difficulties with mess planning and medication when following a carnivorous diet.

Unlike factory- grounded diets, which frequently calculate on simple, minimally reused constituents, rapacious diets may bear further time and trouble to reference high- quality animal products and prepare meals that are both nutritional and satisfying. This can be particularly challenging for those with busy cultures or limited access to fresh, affordable meat and seafood.

Likewise, some persons may witness digestive issues or discomfort when first transitioning to a carnivorous diet. This can be attributed to the unforeseen increase in protein and fat input, as well as the absence of fiber generally set up in factory- grounded foods. Symptoms similar as bloating, constipation, or diarrhea may occur as the body adjusts to its new salutary input, making it important for persons to cover their symptoms and make adaptations as demanded. Despite these difficulties, there are several strategies persons can employ to successfully navigate the transition to a carnivorous diet.

One approach is to gradually transition to a carnivorous diet by sluggishly reducing the input of factory- grounded foods while adding the consumption of animal products. This can help minimize digestive discomfort and allow the body to acclimatize further gradually to its new salutary input.

Another strategy is to prioritize high- quality, nutrient- thick animal products when following a carnivorous diet. This includes choosing lawn- fed beef, pasturage- raised flesh, wild- caught fish, and organic dairy products whenever possible.

By prioritizing nutrient- thick foods, persons can   ensure they're meeting their   nutritive requirements and optimizing their health on a carnivorous   diet.   Mess   planning   and medication are also essential   factors of a successful carnivorous diet.

By planning meals in advance and batch cuisine,   persons can streamline the   cuisine process and ensure they've nutritional meals readily available throughout the week.

Also, incorporating a variety of cuisine styles, similar as grilling, riding, and slow cuisine, can help keep meals intriguing and scrumptious.

Support from like- inclined persons can Also be invaluable when following a carnivorous diet. Whether through online communities, social media groups, or original meetups, connecting with others who partake analogous salutary preferences can give stimulants, alleviation, and practical tips for success.

Also, seeking guidance from healthcare professionals or nutrition experts who are knowledgeable about carnivorous diets can help persons address any enterprises or challenges they may encounter along the way. While embarking on a carnivorous diet may present certain difficulties, with careful planning, perseverance, and support, persons can successfully navigate the transition and experience the implicit benefits of this salutary life. By addressing challenges similar to social pressure, food variety, mess planning, and digestive issues, persons can optimize their health and well- being on a carnivorous diet and enjoy a fulfilling and sustainable way of eating.

Managing Social Coercion

Managing social compulsion when transitioning to a carnivorous diet can be a grueling bid. This salutary choice frequently stands in stark discrepancy to societal morals and can provoke strong responses from friends , family, and indeed nonnatives. Still, with tactfulness, education, and confidence, navigating these social pressures becomes more manageable.

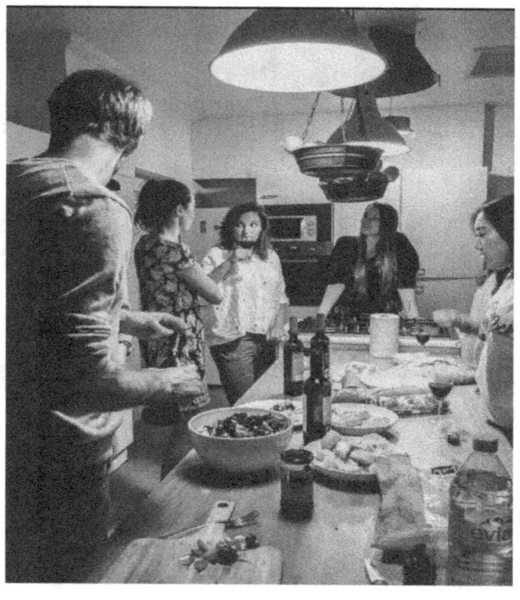

First and foremost, it's pivotal to be confident in your decision and the reasons behind it. Whether you've chosen a carnivorous diet for health reasons, ethical beliefs, or a particular trial,

having a strong understanding of your provocations will help you repel external pressures. Confidence exudes conviction, making it less likely for others to challenge or force you into abandoning your salutary preferences.
Education is another crucial element in managing social compulsion. Be set to explain your salutary choice to others in a clear and terse manner. Share applicable information about the benefits you've endured or the exploration that supports your decision.

 By arming yourself with knowledge, you not only validate your choice but also give others a better understanding of why you've decided on a carnivorous diet. Still, it's essential to approach these exchanges with empathy and understanding. Know that not everyone will partake your perspective or be open to new ideas. Be patient with those who may express dubitation or concern, and avoid getting protective or combative. rather, hear their perspective and address their questions or enterprises calmly and hypocritically. In social settings where food is involved, similar as family gatherings or feasts with friends , navigating salutary differences can be particularly grueling . In these situations, it can be helpful to plan ahead by either offering to bring a dish that aligns with your salutary preferences or communicating your requirements to the host in advance.

By taking a visionary way to ensure your salutary conditions are accommodated, you can minimize implicit discomfort or conflict during mealtime. Likewise, be open to concession and inflexibility when necessary. While sticking to a carnivorous diet may be your preference, there may be instances where accommodating the preferences of others is more conducive to maintaining harmony in social relationships. Finding a balance between honoring your dietary choices and being considerate of others' preferences can help mitigate social coercion.

It's also important to seek out a supportive community of like-minded individuals who can offer guidance, encouragement, and camaraderie on your carnivorous journey. Whether through online forums, social media groups, or local meetups, connecting with others who share similar dietary beliefs can provide a sense of belonging and validation, especially during moments of social pressure.

Ultimately, managing social coercion when embarking on a carnivorous diet requires a combination of confidence, education, empathy, and flexibility. By staying true to your convictions, communicating effectively, and seeking support from a supportive community, you can navigate social pressures with grace and resilience. Remember, your dietary choices are personal, and it's essential to prioritize your health and well-being above external opinions or expectations.

Handling Intense Wants
Embarking on a carnivorous diet can indeed stir up intense desires, especially if you're

accustomed to a more varied eating plan. Here are a few tips to handle those cravings:

1. Stay Focused on Goals:
Remind yourself why you chose this diet in the first place. Whether it's for health reasons or personal experimentation, keeping your goals in mind can help you stay motivated.

2. Experiment with Recipes:
Explore different cooking methods and recipes within the constraints of your diet. This can add variety and excitement to your meals, making it easier to stick with your plan.

3. Find Support:
Connect with others who are following a similar diet for encouragement and advice. Online communities and forums can be valuable resources for sharing experiences and strategies for dealing with cravings.

4. Practice Mindfulness:

When cravings strike, take a moment to acknowledge them without judgment. Then, focus on the physical sensations in your body and engage in an activity to distract yourself until the craving passes.

5. Stay Hydrated:

Sometimes, feelings of hunger can be mistaken for thirst. Drinking water throughout the day can help keep cravings at bay.

6. Plan Ahead:

Make sure you have plenty of carnivore-friendly foods available to prevent feeling deprived. Stock up on meats, eggs, and other protein sources so you always have options on hand.

7. Seek Professional Guidance:

If you're struggling to manage intense cravings or find the diet unsustainable, consider consulting a healthcare professional or registered dietitian who can offer personalized advice and support.

CHAPTER 6

Exercise and Health

Embarking on a carnivorous diet, which focuses exclusively on the consumption of animal products, is a significant shift from more balanced or plant-inclusive dietary approaches. This diet, Also known as the carnivore diet, often includes meat, fish, eggs, and some dairy products. The rationale behind this diet is that it mirrors the dietary patterns of our ancestors and aims to eliminate potential dietary triggers for chronic diseases and inflammation. When combined with exercise, the carnivorous diet presents unique considerations and benefits for health and fitness. This essay will explore the implications of this diet on exercise performance, body composition, metabolic health, and overall well-being.

Exercise Performance on a Carnivorous Diet

Exercise performance is a critical area to examine when considering the carnivorous diet. This diet is inherently low in carbohydrates, which are traditionally considered the primary energy source for high-intensity activities. Instead, the body relies heavily on fats and proteins for energy. This metabolic shift can have several effects on physical performance.

1. Adaptation Period

Initially, individuals may experience a decline in exercise performance as the body adapts to using fat as the primary fuel source. This phase, often referred to as "keto flu" in ketogenic diets, can involve symptoms like fatigue, headaches, and irritability. For athletes, this adaptation period can be particularly challenging, but it usually resolves within a few weeks as the body becomes more efficient at burning fat.

2. Endurance Exercise

For endurance activities such as long-distance running or cycling, a carnivorous diet can be beneficial. Once fat-adapted, the body can access a virtually limitless energy supply from body fat stores, enhancing stamina and reducing the need for frequent carbohydrate refueling. Some endurance athletes report improved performance and recovery times on a carnivore diet.

3. Strength and Power

High-intensity, anaerobic activities like weightlifting or sprinting traditionally rely on glycogen stored in muscles. While there may be concerns about reduced performance in these areas due to lower glycogen availability, many practitioners of the carnivorous diet report maintaining or even improving their strength and power. This could be attributed to the high protein intake supporting muscle repair and growth.

Body Composition and Weight Management

The carnivorous diet can significantly impact body composition and weight management, often leading to fat loss and muscle preservation or gain.

1. Fat Loss
The high protein content of the diet can promote satiety and reduce overall caloric intake, aiding in weight loss. Additionally, the low carbohydrate intake leads to lower insulin levels, promoting fat burning. Some individuals on the carnivore diet experience rapid and substantial weight loss, especially in the initial stages.

2. Muscle Mass
Adequate protein intake is crucial for muscle maintenance and growth. The carnivorous diet, with its emphasis on meat, provides a rich source of high-quality protein. This can be particularly beneficial for those engaging in resistance training or other forms of exercise aimed at building muscle mass.

3. Metabolic Efficiency

Over time, individuals on a carnivore diet may experience increased metabolic efficiency. By relying on fat as the primary energy source, the body becomes better at utilizing stored fat for energy, potentially leading to a leaner physique and enhanced overall metabolic health.

Metabolic Health

The carnivorous diet can have profound effects on metabolic health, influencing factors such as blood sugar control, cholesterol levels, and inflammation.

1. Blood Sugar Control

With virtually no carbohydrate intake, the carnivore diet can stabilize blood sugar levels and reduce insulin resistance. This can be particularly salutary for persons with type 2 diabetes or metabolic pattern. numerous votaries report better blood glucose situations and a reduced need for drugs.

2. Cholesterol and Heart Health

The impact of the carnivorous diet on cholesterol situations is complex and can vary among persons. Some people may see an increase in LDL cholesterol, while others witness advancements in HDL cholesterol and triglyceride situations. The diet's effects on heart health are still debated , but some exploration suggests that it may ameliorate labels of cardiovascular health by reducing inflammation and perfecting lipid biographies.

3. Inflammation

Habitual inflammation is linked to multitudinous health issues, including heart complaint, arthritis, and autoimmune conditions. The carnivore diet eliminates numerous common seditious foods, similar as refined sugars, grains, and seed canvases , which can lead to a reduction in systemic inflammation. numerous people on this diet report advancements in seditious labels and symptom relief for colorful habitual conditions.

Overall Well- being

Beyond the physical goods, the carnivorous diet can   impact overall well- being, including internal health and cognitive function.

1. Mental Clarity and Mood

Some votaries report enhanced internal clarity, focus, and mood stability on a carnivore diet. This may be due to stabilized blood sugar situations, reduced inflammation, and the elimination of salutary triggers for internal health issues. High- quality proteins and fats support brain health, which could contribute to these cognitive benefits.

2. Energy situations

Once the body adapts to the diet, numerous persons witness stable and sustained energy situations throughout the day. This is in discrepancy to the energy oscillations frequently associated with carbohydrate-rich diets.

3. Digestive Health The carnivorous diet can ameliorate digestive health by barring foods that

generally beget digestive issues, similar as fiber, gluten, and other factory- grounded antinutrients. Still, some persons may witness digestive adaptations when starting the diet, including changes in bowel habits.

Considerations and Implicit downsides

While the carnivorous diet offers colorful benefits, there are implicit downsides and considerations to keep in mind.

1. Nutrient Deficiency

The elimination of factory foods raises enterprises about implicit nutrient scarcities, particularly in vitamins C and E, fiber, and certain phytonutrients. persons on this diet need to ensure they're carrying all necessary nutrients from animal sources, conceivably through organ flesh and supplementation.

2. Sustainability and Variety

The restrictive nature of the diet can make it grueling to maintain in the long term. Lack of variety might lead to salutary tedium and make it harder to cleave to the diet.

3. Social and Practical Challenges
Clinging to a carnivore diet can be socially and virtually grueling , particularly in social situations and when dining out. It requires careful planning and commitment.

The carnivorous diet, when combined with exercise, can offer multitudinous benefits, including better body composition, enhanced metabolic health, and better overall well- being. Still, it's essential to approach this diet with a clear understanding of its implicit challenges and the need for careful planning to insure nutritive acceptability. As with any diet, individual responses can vary, and it may be salutary to consult with a healthcare professional before making significant salutary changes.

By considering these factors, persons can make informed opinions about whether the carnivore diet aligns with their health and fitness pretensions.

Carnivore Exercise Advice: Maintaining Nutritional Balance

Embarking on a carnivorous diet while maintaining an active life requires careful consideration of nutritive balance to support exercise performance and overall health.

The carnivore diet, which emphasizes the consumption of animal products simply, is innately different from further conventional diets that include a variety of food groups.

This essay will give comprehensive advice for maintaining nutritive balance while engaging in regular physical exertion on a carnivore diet.

The carnivore diet is primarily composed of meat, fish, eggs, and some dairy products. It excludes all factory- grounded foods, including fruits, vegetables, grains, nuts, and seeds. The explanation behind this diet is that it aligns more closely with the salutary patterns of our ancestors, potentially offering benefits similar to reduced inflammation, better metabolic health, and enhanced internal clarity.

Still, this diet's restrictive nature necessitates careful planning to avoid nutrient scarcity, especially for those who exercise regularly.

Protein Input and Muscle conservation
Protein is a foundation of the carnivore diet, and its part in muscle conservation and form is pivotal, particularly for those engaging in regular physical exertion.

1. Acceptable Protein Consumption

Athletes and active persons have advanced protein conditions to support muscle form and growth. It's generally recommended to consume between 1.2 to2.2 grams of protein per kilogram of body weight per day. On a carnivore diet, this is fluently attainable through the consumption of colorful animal proteins similar to beef, pork, flesh, fish, and eggs.

2. Variety of Protein Sources
While muscle meat is a primary protein source, incorporating a variety of animal proteins ensures a broader diapason of amino acids and

other nutrients. Including fish, especially adipose fish like salmon, provides essential omega- 3 adipose acids that are salutary for cardiovascular health and inflammation reduction.

Fats for Energy and Nutrient immersion
Fats play a pivotal part in a carnivorous diet, serving as the primary energy source due to the low carbohydrate input.

1. Incorporating Healthy Fats
To ensure sufficient energy situations, especially for abidance conditioning, include healthy fats from sources like adipose cuts of meat, adulation, ghee, tallow, and adipose fish. These fats not only give energy but Also aid in the immersion of fat-answerable vitamins(A, D, E, and K).

2. Balance Saturated and Unsaturated Fats
While animal fats are high in impregnated fats, it's important to balance these with unsaturated fats to support heart health. Incorporating

further fish and using fats like ghee and tallow can help achieve this balance.

Vitamins and Minerals Avoiding scarcities One of the main enterprises with a carnivore diet is the eventuality for nutrient scarcities, particularly in vitamins and minerals generally sourced from factory- grounded foods.

1. Vitamin C

Although the carnivore diet can give some vitamin C through organ flesh, similar to liver and order, it might still be lower than a diet that includes fruits and vegetables. Some votaries calculate on the small quantities present in raw or minimally cooked flesh. icing the addition of organ flesh can help alleviate this threat.

2. Magnesium

Magnesium is less abundant in animal foods compared to factory foods. Active persons, especially those engaging in violent exercise, might need to consider supplements to meet their magnesium conditions for muscle function and recovery.

3. Potassium analogous to magnesium

Potassium is pivotal for muscle function and overall health. Foods like adipose fish and organ flesh contain some potassium, but supplementation might be necessary for those not meeting their requirements through diet alone.

4. Calcium

While dairy products give calcium, those avoiding dairy on a carnivore diet should consider bone- in fish or bone broth as indispensable sources. Also, icing sufficient vitamin D input through exposure to sun or supplementation can promote calcium immersion.

Hydration and Electrolyte Balance

Hydration and maintaining electrolyte balance are critical, especially for those engaging in regular exercise.

1. Sodium The carnivore diet can be naturally low in sodium due to the absence of reused

foods. Still, active persons lose sodium through sweat and need to   insure acceptable input to maintain electrolyte balance. Adding swab to meals and drinking electrolyte- enhanced water can help help imbalances.

2. Hydration Acceptable hydration is essential for exercise performance and recovery. Drinking water regularly throughout the day and consuming electrolyte-rich broths can help maintain hydration status.

Timing and Composition
Strategically planning mess timing and composition can optimize exercise performance and recovery.

1. Pre-Workout Nutrition
Consuming a mess rich in protein and moderate in fat 1- 2 hours before a drill can give sustained energy. For high- intensity conditioning, some may profit from a lower, fluently digestible protein source like eggs or a protein shake.

2. Post-Workout Nutrition

Post-workout meals should concentrate on replenishing nutrients and supporting muscle recovery. A mess containing a significant portion of protein along with healthy fats can help repair muscle towel and restore energy situations.

3. Intermittent Fasting

Some persons on a carnivore diet practice intermittent fasting, which can align with their exercise routines.

However, it's pivotal to ensure that nutrient input during eating windows is sufficient to support overall health and exercise demands, If choosing to gormandize.

Monitoring Health and Performance

Regularly covering health labels and exercise performance is vital to insure the carnivore diet is meeting an existent's requirements.

1. Blood Tests

Periodic blood tests can help track nutrient situations, similar as vitamin D, B12, iron, and electrolytes, allowing for adaptations in diet or supplementation as demanded.

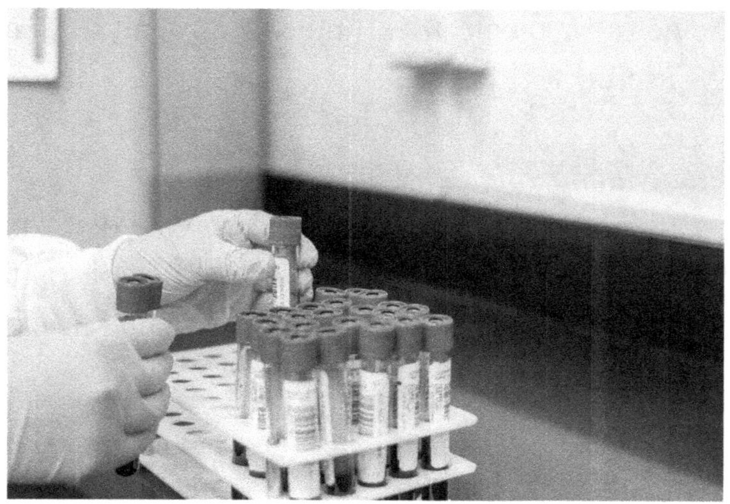

2. Performance Metrics

Keeping track of exercise performance, including strength, abidance, and recovery times, can give perceptivity into how well the diet is supporting physical exertion. Any significant declines might indicate the need for salutary adaptations.

3. Body Composition Monitoring body composition changes, similar to muscle mass and fat chance, can help ensure that the diet supports fitness pretensions. Tools like body reviews or bioelectrical impedance analysis can be useful.

Individualization and Inflexibility
Individual responses to the carnivore diet can vary, and it's essential to remain flexible and make adaptations grounded on particular health and performance.

1.Substantiated Approach
What works for one person may not work for another. It's important to   listen to one's body and acclimate to the diet consequently. This might involve tweaking protein and fat rates, incorporating supplements, or modifying mess timing.

2. Consulting Professionals   Working with a healthcare provider or a nutritionist familiar with the carnivore diet can   give   substantiated guidance and help address any nutritive gaps or health enterprises.

Maintaining nutritive balance while following a carnivore diet and engaging in regular exercise requires careful planning and attention to detail. By   icing acceptable protein and fat input, addressing implicit nutrient   scarcities, maintaining hydration and electrolyte balance, and strategically timing   meals,   persons can support their exercise performance and overall health. Regular monitoring and a flexible approach are   crucial to achieving long- term success on this diet. With the right strategies in place, the carnivore diet can be compatible with an active life, offering benefits similar to better body composition, enhanced metabolic health, and better overall well- being.

CHAPTER 7

Troubleshooting

Troubleshooting the Carnivorous Diet

The carnivorous diet, focusing only on animal products like meat, fish, eggs, and some dairy, can offer many health benefits but Also presents unique challenges. This guide will help you troubleshoot common issues to ensure you maintain a healthy and balanced approach.

1. Adapting to the Diet

Problem: During the first few weeks, you might experience "keto flu" symptoms like fatigue, headaches, and irritability.

Solution:
- Hydration: Drink plenty of water.
- Electrolytes: Supplement with sodium, potassium, and magnesium. Add salt to your meals and drink broth.

- Gradual Transition: If symptoms are severe, reduce carbs slowly instead of cutting them all at once.

2. Digestive Issues

Problem: Common issues include constipation, diarrhea, and bloating.

Solution:
- Constipation: Drink more water and increase fat intake. Bone broth and fatty meats can help.
- Diarrhea: Gradually increase fat consumption to help your body adjust. Ensure meats are well-cooked.
- Bloating: Eat smaller meals more frequently and reduce dairy if it causes issues.

3. Nutrient Deficiencies

Problem: Potential deficiencies in vitamins and minerals like vitamin C, magnesium, and potassium.

Solution:

- Vitamin C: Include organ meats like liver and kidney.

- Magnesium and Potassium: Consider supplements if needed. Fatty fish and bone broth can help.

- Fiber: Many find they don't need fiber on this diet, but if needed, consider small, targeted supplements.

4. Energy Levels and Exercise

Problem: Reduced energy and performance due to low carbs.

Solution:

- Fat Adaptation: It may take several weeks for your body to adjust.

- Meal Timing: Eat a protein and fat-rich meal a couple of hours before exercise. Post-workout, have a nutrient-dense meal.

- Adjust Workouts: Reduce intensity during the adaptation phase and increase it gradually.

5. Weight Plateaus

Problem: Stalled weight loss after initial success.

Solution:
- Caloric Intake: Track your food to ensure you're in a caloric deficit if weight loss is your goal.
- Meal Frequency: Try intermittent fasting to overcome plateaus.
- Exercise: Mix cardio and strength training to boost metabolism.

6. Cravings and Emotional Eating

Problem: Strong cravings for carbs and sweets.

Solution:
- High-Fat Snacks: Satisfy cravings with pork rinds, cheese, or eggs.
- Stay Full: Eat enough protein and fat at meals.

- Stress Management: Use mindfulness, meditation, or hobbies to manage emotional eating.

7. Social and Practical Challenges

Problem: Difficulty in social situations and dining out.

Solution:
- Planning: Check menus ahead of time or eat before events. Bring your own meat-based dishes.
- Communication: Explain your dietary choices to friends and family.
- Adaptability: Choose meat-centric restaurants and ask for modifications.

8. Sustainability

Problem: Difficulty maintaining the diet long-term due to its restrictive nature.

Solution:
- Variety: Try different types of meat, fish, and organ meats. Experiment with cooking methods and recipes.
- Support Systems: Engage with online communities or find local groups for support.
- Listen to Your Body: Make necessary adjustments based on your body's responses.

9. Medical Concerns

Problem: Pre-existing conditions or adverse health effects.

Solution:
- Regular Monitoring: Get regular blood tests and health check-ups.
- Professional Guidance: Consult a healthcare provider familiar with the diet for personalized advice.

The carnivorous diet can be beneficial but requires careful planning to avoid common pitfalls. By addressing issues like digestive problems, nutrient deficiencies, energy levels, weight plateaus, cravings, social challenges, and sustainability, you can successfully navigate this diet. Always listen to your body and seek professional guidance when needed to maintain a healthy and balanced approach.

Typical Errors and Their Fixes Knowing When to Ask for Assistance

The carnivorous diet, which focuses exclusively on animal products such as meat, fish, eggs, and some dairy, is a straightforward yet restrictive dietary approach. While many find success with this way of eating, it is not uncommon to encounter obstacles. Understanding common errors and knowing when to seek help can make a significant difference in achieving your health goals. This guide outlines typical errors on the carnivorous diet and their fixes, emphasizing the importance of asking for assistance when needed.

1. Inadequate Protein and Fat Intake

Error: Consuming insufficient amounts of protein and fat, leading to fatigue, muscle loss, and overall energy deficiency.

Fix:
- Increase Protein Intake: Ensure you are consuming enough high-quality animal protein. Aim for 1.2 to 2.2 grams of protein per kilogram of body weight daily.
- Add Healthy Fats: Incorporate more healthy animal fats into your diet. Opt for fatty cuts of meat, butter, ghee, and fatty fish like salmon.
- Balance Ratios: Balance your macronutrient ratios to ensure you are getting enough calories from fat to sustain energy levels.

When to Ask for Assistance: If you're unsure about your macronutrient needs or experience persistent fatigue, consider consulting a nutritionist or dietitian familiar with the carnivorous diet.

2. Ignoring Electrolyte Balance

Error: Failing to maintain proper electrolyte balance, resulting in symptoms such as headaches, muscle cramps, and fatigue.

Fix:
-     Supplement   Electrolytes: Regularly supplement with sodium, potassium, and magnesium. Adding salt to meals, drinking bone broth, and considering magnesium supplements can help.
- Hydrate Properly: Drink plenty of water to stay hydrated, especially if you are active and lose electrolytes through sweat.

When to Ask for Assistance: If you experience severe symptoms like persistent muscle cramps or headaches, seek advice from a healthcare professional who can recommend appropriate electrolyte supplementation.

3. Monotony in Diet

Error: Eating a limited variety of animal products, leading to potential nutrient deficiencies and diet fatigue.

Fix:
- Diversify Protein Sources: Include a variety of meats such as beef, pork, poultry, lamb, and fish. Incorporate organ meats like liver and kidney for additional nutrients.
- Explore Different Cooking Methods: Use different cooking techniques like grilling, roasting, slow-cooking, and broiling to keep meals interesting.
- Include Dairy Carefully: If you tolerate dairy, include cheese, butter, and cream for variety and additional nutrients.
When to Ask for Assistance: If you struggle to create diverse meals or feel unmotivated by your food choices, consulting a nutritionist for meal planning ideas can be beneficial.

4. Undervaluing the Adaptation Period

Error : Awaiting immediate results and undervaluing the time it takes for the body to acclimatize to the carnivorous diet, leading to despondency.

 Fix:
-- Be Case Understand that the body needs time to acclimatize to a new energy source. This period can last several weeks.
- Examiner Progress Keep track of changes in your energy situations, mood, and physical performance to stay motivated.
-Gradual Transition. If symptoms are severe, consider gradually reducing carbohydrates rather than barring them suddenly.

 When to Ask for backing
 If you feel persistently bad or are doubtful about your progress, seek guidance from a healthcare provider to insure you're conforming healthily.

5. Miisruling Digestive Issues

Error: Ignoring or misleading common digestive issues similar as constipation, diarrhea, and bloating.

Fix:

- Acclimate Fat Intake. Increase or drop fat input grounded on your digestive response. For constipation, further fat may help for diarrhea, reducing fat can be salutary.
- Stay Doused. Drink plenty of water to prop digestion and help constipation.
- Introduce Foods sluggishly. When trying new animal products, introduce them sluggishly to cover how your body reacts. When to Ask for backing If digestive issues persist or worsen, it's important to consult a healthcare professional to rule out underpinning conditions and admit acclimatized advice.

6. Shy Nutrient Input.

Error: threat of nutrient scarcities due to the rejection of factory- grounded foods.

 Fix:
- Incorporate Organ Flesh Include nutrient- thick organ flesh regularly to gain vitamins and minerals not as abundant in muscle flesh
. - Consider Supplements. If necessary, use supplements for vitamins and minerals like vitamin C, magnesium, and potassium.
- Examiner Health Labels Regularly check blood situations for crucial nutrients to insure you aren't deficient
.

When to Ask for backing.
If you suspect nutrient scarcities or experience symptoms similar to fatigue, weakness, or poor vulnerable function, consult a healthcare provider for applicable testing and supplementation advice.

7. Handling Social and Practical Challenges

Error: floundering with social situations and practicality, leading to passions of insulation or difficulty maintaining the diet.

 Fix:
-Plan Ahead When attending social events, plan your meals in advance or bring your own carnivore-friendly options.
  - Communicate requirements Explain your salutary requirements to friends and family to gain their support and understanding.
- Find Support Join online communities or original groups of people following the carnivorous diet for tips and stimulants.

When to Ask for backing
If social challenges come inviting or lead to salutary non-compliance, seeking support from a counselor or dietitian can help you develop strategies to navigate these situations.

8. Lack of Monitoring and Adjustment

Error: Failing to regularly cover progress and make necessary adaptations, leading to sour results.

Fix:

- Track Your Progress Keep a journal of your food input, physical performance, and health labels to identify trends and make adaptations.
- Acclimate as demanded. Be flexible and willing to tweak your diet based on how your body responds. This may include altering mess frequency, portion sizes, or the types of animal products you consume.

When to Ask for backing

Still, consulting a nutritionist can give substantiated guidance, If you're doubtful about how to acclimate your diet or if you aren't seeing the asked results.

The carnivorous diet can offer multitudinous health benefits, but it isn't without its challenges. Common crimes similar to shy nutrient input, electrolyte imbalances, and digestive issues can be managed with careful planning and adaptations. Knowing when to seek professional backing is pivotal for addressing patient problems and icing long- term success. By staying informed, covering your progress, and seeking help when necessary, you can navigate the carnivorous diet effectively and achieve your health pretensions.

CHAPTER 8

Durable Achievements

Durable Achievement on Embarking on a Rapacious Diet

 The carnivorous diet, constantly pertained to as the carnivore diet, has gained popularity as an extreme form of low- carbohydrate eating. Its premise is simple: consume only animal products and count all plant- predicated foods. Proponents claim that this diet can lead to numerous health benefits, including weight loss, bettered internal clarity, and relief from habitual ails. Still, achieving and maintaining success on a carnivorous diet requires careful planning, a deep understanding of nutritional conditions, and a commitment to sustainability.

This essay explores the way and considerations necessary to achieve durable success on a carnivorous diet. The carnivorous diet is principally an elimination diet that focuses simply on animal - predicated foods. This includes meat, fish, eggs, and some dairy products. All plant- predicated foods, including fruits, vegetables, grains, nuts, and seeds, are barred.

The idea is that mortal beings are optimally designed to thrive on animal products and that multitudinous modern affections stem from the consumption of plant- predicated foods.

Health Benefits and Challenges

Proponents of the carnivorous diet argue that it can lead to significant health advancements. These benefits are constantly attributed to the high protein and fat content, which can promote malnutrition and reduce overall calorie input.

Also, barring carbohydrates can stabilize blood sugar situations and potentially reduce inflammation. Still, transitioning to and maintaining a carnivorous diet can pose challenges. One significant concern is the eventuality for nutrient deficiencies, particularly in vitamins and minerals generally set up in plant foods, analogous as vitamin C, magnesium, and potassium.

Another challenge is the social and cultural aspect of eating. The diet is largely restrictive, making it delicate to partake in social events and dine out.

Ways To Achieve Success

1. Education and Planning

Before embarking on a carnivorous diet, it's vital to educate oneself about the nutritional conditions and implicit pitfalls. Understanding the wisdom behind the diet, including how to source nutrient-thick animal products and the physiological goods of such a restrictive authority, is essential. Planning meals and icing a variety of animal foods can help palliate the trouble of nutrient deficiencies.

2. Gradual Transition

For those acquainted with a diet rich in carbohydrates and plant- predicated foods, an unlooked-for shift to a each- meat diet can be unmanning. A gradual transition can help the body adapt to the increased fat and protein input while minimizing implicit digestive issues. Starting with a ketogenic or low- carb diet before fully committing to the carnivorous diet can ease this transition.

3. Nutrient-thick

Choosing fastening on nutrient-thick animal products is critical. While muscle meat like steak and funk are millions, incorporating organ meat analogous as liver and order can give essential vitamins and minerals. Bone broth is another precious addition, offering collagen and other salutary mixes.

4. Monitoring Health

Regular monitoring of health markers is essential to ensure that the diet is salutary and not causing detriment. Blood tests can track cholesterol situations, nutrient status, and markers of inflammation. Working with a healthcare provider knowledgeable about the carnivorous diet can give substantiated guidance and acclimations.

5. Community and Support

Engaging with a community of like- inclined persons can give support and provocation. Online forums, social media groups, and original meetups can offer a wealth of information, share exploits, and help troubleshoot common issues. Support from family and buddies can also make the salutary shift more sustainable.

Implicit pitfalls and results

1. Nutrient deficiencies

One of the main examples of the carnivorous diet is the trouble of nutrient deficiencies. While animal products are rich in multitudinous nutrients, they warrant others that are generally set up in plant foods. For illustration, vitamin C, generally associated with fruits and vegetables, is vital for collagen emulsion and vulnerable function. To palliate this, some carnivore diet followers incorporate organ meat, which contain small amounts of vitamin C, and emphasize the consumption of fresh, minimally reused meat.

2. Digestive Issues

An unlooked-for increase in fat input can lead to digestive issues analogous as diarrhea, constipation, and bloating. To address this, it's judicious to increase fat input gradually and ensure a balance of different types of fats. Including bone broth and gelatin can support gut health and meliorate digestion.

3. Social and Cerebral Factors

The restrictive nature of the carnivorous diet can lead to heartstrings of sequestration, especially in social situations centered around food. Developing strategies to handle social events, analogous as eating beforehand or bringing one's own food, can help. Also, fastening on the reasons for choosing the diet and the health benefits it provides can strengthen decisiveness.

Long- Term Sustainability

Achieving long- term success on a carnivorous diet requires a sustainable approach. This involves regular tone- assessment and acclimations as demanded.

Also are some strategies for long- term adherence

1. Strictness and Adaptation

While strict adherence is necessary for some persons, others may benefit from occasional strictness. Incorporating small amounts of low- bane plant foods, like certain fruits ornon- stiff vegetables, can give variety and fresh nutrients without significantly compromising the principles of the diet.

2. Continuous Knowledge

Staying informed about new disquisition and developments in the field of nutrition can help upgrade the diet and ensure it remains optimal. Engaging with the broader health and wholesomeness community can give new perceptivity and help recession.

3. Personalization

No single diet fits everyone perfectly. Personalizing the carnivorous diet to fit one's unique health conditions, life, and preferences can enhance sustainability. This might involve conforming macronutrient rates, trying different types of animal products, or incorporating supplements if necessary.

4. Mental Health and Wellbeing

A holistic approach to health includes internal well- being. Engaging in conditioning that promotes internal health, similar to exercise, contemplation, and pursuits, can round the salutary changes and ameliorate overall quality of life.

Achieving durable success involves a comprehensive approach that includes education, careful planning, and nonstop monitoring. By addressing implicit risks and conforming the diet to individual requirements, it's possible to maintain this diet long- term and enjoy its benefits.

Community support and a focus on overall well-being further enhance the sustainability of this diet. As with any significant salutary change, it's judicious to consult with healthcare professionals to knitter the approach to one's specific health requirements and conditions.

Making a Life of Carnivory Extended Fasts and Sustainable Intermittent Fasting

The carnivorous diet, characterized by exclusive consumption of animal - grounded foods, has garnered attention for its implicit health benefits. When paired with fasting protocols, similar as extended fasting and intermittent fasting(IF), it can potentially enhance these benefits. Integrating fasting into a rapacious life involves understanding the community between the diet and fasting, planning for sustainability, and addressing implicit challenges.

This essay explores how to make a life of carnivory amended with extended fasts and sustainable intermittent fasting.   The Carnivorous Diet The carnivorous diet is a form of extreme low- carb, high- protein eating that eliminates all factory- grounded foods. The diet focuses solely on animal products like meat, fish, eggs, and some dairy. lawyers argue that it aligns with   mortal evolutionary history, potentially reducing inflammation, perfecting internal clarity, and abetting in weight loss.

The part of Fasting

Fasting, the voluntary abstention from food for a set period, has been rehearsed for glories for both religious and health reasons. Recent scientific studies punctuate the benefits of fasting, which include enhanced metabolic health, better insulin perceptivity, and autophagy(the body's process of drawing out damaged cells).

Fasting protocols can be astronomically distributed into extended fasting and intermittent fasting.

* Extended Fasting

Extended fasting refers to ages of no food input for 24 hours or further. This type of fasting can range from one day to several days. Extended fasting is believed to give profound health benefits by allowing the body to enter deeper countries of ketosis, autophagy, and cellular form.

*Intermittent Fasting   Intermittent fasting(IF) involves cycling between ages of eating and dieting within a 24- hour period. Common styles include the 16/8 system(16 hours of fasting and an 8- hour eating window), the 52 system(eating typically for five days and significantly reducing calorie input for two non-consecutive days), and the Eat- Stop- Eat system(24- hour fasts formerly or doubly a week).

Combining Carnivory and Fasting

Combining a carnivorous diet with fasting protocols can potentially amplify the benefits of both practices. The high- fat, high- protein nature of the carnivorous diet helps sustain energy situations during fasting ages, making it easier to cleave to fasting schedules.

Benefits of the Combination

1. Enhanced Ketosis

Both fasting and a carnivorous diet promote ketosis, a metabolic state where the body burns fat for energy rather than carbohydrates. Enhanced ketosis can lead to bettered weight operation, internal clarity, and sustained energy situations.

2. Bettered Insulin perceptivity

The reduction in carbohydrate input from the carnivorous diet, combined with the insulin-regulating goods of fasting, can significantly ameliorate insulin perceptivity, reducing the threat of type 2 diabetes.

3. Accelerated Autophagy

Fasting accelerates autophagy, helping the body to clean out damaged cells and regenerate new bones . The nutrient- thick, poison-free nature of animal products can support this cellular revivification process.

4. Digestive Health

 The carnivorous diet is frequently touted for its simplicity and ease on the digestive system. When paired with fasting, it can give the digestive system ample time to rest and recover, potentially easing issues like bloating and inflammation.

Enforcing Fasting in a Rapacious life

-Starting with Intermittent Fasting .

 For those new to fasting, starting with intermittent fasting can be more manageable. The 16/8 system is a popular starting point. This involves fasting for 16 hours(including sleep time) and eating within an 8- hour window.

For illustration, one might eat between noon and 8 PM and presto from 8 PM to noon the coming day.

-Transitioning to Extended Fasting.
Once comfortable with intermittent fasting, one can gradually incorporate extended fasts. Start with a 24- hour presto, maybe from regale one day to regale the coming. As the body adapts, longer fasts can be tried, but it's pivotal to hear to the body and ensure acceptable hydration and electrolyte balance.

-Meal Planning and Preparation
Planning meals around nutrient- thick animal products is crucial. During eating windows, concentrate on a variety of flesh, fish, eggs, and organ flesh to ensure a broad diapason of nutrients. Bone broth can be particularly salutary for its collagen content and gut- mending parcels.

-Hydration and Electrolytes Staying doused and maintaining electrolyte balance is critical during fasting. Water, herbal teas, and electrolyte supplements(sodium, potassium, magnesium) can help dehumidification and electrolyte imbalances, which are common during extended fasts.

-Sustainability and Challenges

An implicit challenge of combining a carnivorous diet with fasting is icing nutritive acceptability. While animal products are rich in numerous essential nutrients, it's important to consume a variety of them to help scarcities. Regularly including organ flesh, bone broth, and adipose fish can help cover most nutritive bases.

- Social and Cerebral Aspects

The restrictive nature of a carnivorous diet and the discipline needed for fasting can be socially segregating. Chancing a probative community, either online or in person, can help sustain provocation and adherence. Being transparent with friends and family about salutary choices can also grease social situations.

-Monitoring Health   Regular health check- ups are essential to cover the body's response to this life. Blood tests can help track cholesterol situations, blood sugar, and nutrient status. Working with a healthcare provider knowledgeable about both carnivory and fasting can give acclimatized guidance..

Long-Term Strategies for Success

-Flexibility and Adaptation

Rigid adherence to any diet can lead to burnout. Building flexibility into the fasting schedule and being open to occasional dietary variations can enhance long-term sustainability. For instance, incorporating occasional carbohydrate refeeds or plant-based foods might be beneficial for some individuals.

-Continuous Learning and Adjustment

Staying informed about new research and developments in nutrition and fasting is crucial.

Regularly assessing one's health and adjusting the diet and fasting protocols as needed can help maintain balance and prevent potential issues.

-Mental and Physical Well-being

A holistic approach to health includes mental and physical well-being. Incorporating regular physical activity, stress management techniques like meditation or yoga, and ensuring adequate sleep can complement the dietary and fasting regimen.

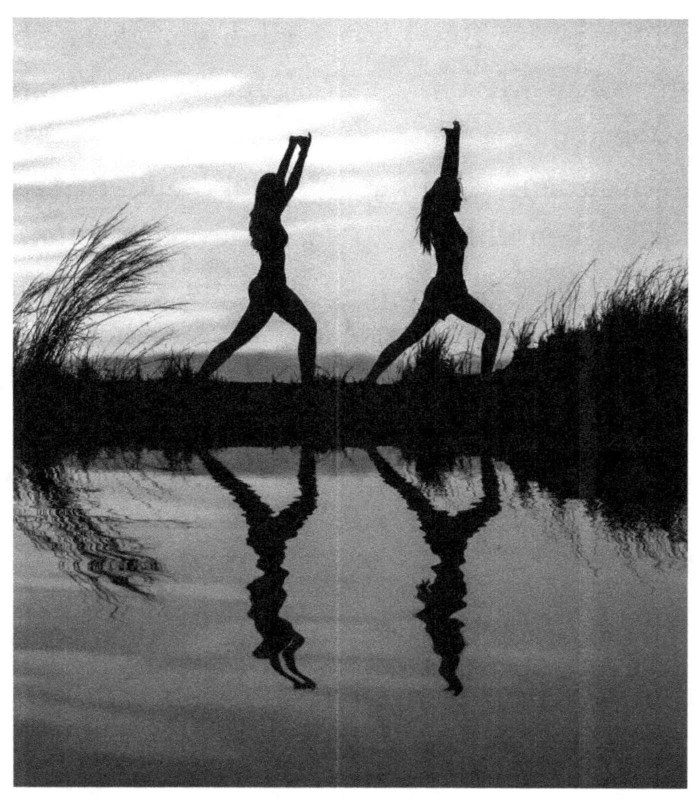

Making a life of carnivory enriched with extended fasts and sustainable intermittent fasting involves a multifaceted approach. Understanding the benefits and potential challenges of both practices, planning meals carefully, maintaining hydration and electrolyte balance, and regularly monitoring health are crucial steps. Building flexibility and support into the lifestyle can enhance long-term sustainability.

As with any significant dietary and lifestyle change, consulting with healthcare professionals to tailor the approach to individual needs and conditions is advisable. By thoughtfully integrating these practices, one can potentially achieve significant health benefits and maintain them over the long term.

CONCLUSION

Appreciating Your Carnivorous Experience, Hoping for a Healthier Future

In a world overflowing with dietary advice and nutritional fads, the carnivorous diet stands out as a unique and often controversial approach. Rooted in the consumption of animal products exclusively, this diet challenges conventional wisdom by eliminating all plant-based foods. As you embark on or continue your carnivorous journey, it's important to reflect on the experience and envision the healthier future it promises. Here's a closer look at how to appreciate your carnivorous lifestyle and maintain a hopeful outlook for your well-being.

For many, the initial phase of the carnivorous diet can be transformative. The simplicity of the diet eliminates the guesswork from meal planning, and many find that their cravings for sugar and carbs diminish significantly. The focus on nutrient-dense animal products can lead to noticeable improvements in energy levels, mental clarity, and overall mood. This phase is often marked by a newfound sense of control and satisfaction with food choices, setting a positive tone for the journey ahead.

One of the most compelling aspects of the carnivorous diet is its potential health benefits. Many adherents report significant weight loss, improved insulin sensitivity, and reduced inflammation. Conditions such as autoimmune disorders, digestive issues, and chronic pain have been known to improve, providing a powerful testament to the diet's efficacy. By focusing on these health gains, you can stay motivated and committed to your carnivorous path.

The carnivorous diet simplifies nutrition in a profound way. By consuming only animal products, you eliminate the need to balance macronutrients meticulously. The high-protein, high-fat composition of the diet promotes satiety, making it easier to maintain a caloric deficit if weight loss is a goal. The absence of processed foods and sugars reduces the risk of overeating, leading to more consistent and sustainable dietary habits.

While the carnivorous diet may seem restrictive, it offers a unique opportunity to appreciate the rich flavors and textures of animal products. From succulent steaks and juicy burgers to savory roasts and tender fish, the variety within the carnivorous spectrum is impressive. Exploring different cuts of meat, experimenting with various cooking techniques, and savoring the natural flavors of high-quality animal products can turn each meal into a culinary delight.

Embarking on a carnivorous journey can sometimes feel isolating, given its deviation from mainstream dietary norms. However, the growing community of carnivorous diet enthusiasts offers a valuable support network. Engaging with like-minded individuals through social media, forums, and local meetups can provide encouragement, share tips and recipes, and help troubleshoot any challenges. This sense of community fosters a collective appreciation of the lifestyle and reinforces the commitment to a healthier future.

No diet is without its challenges, and the carnivorous diet is no exception. Potential obstacles such as social pressures, dining out, and occasional cravings can arise. However, by staying focused on the positive changes you've experienced and the health benefits you're working towards, these challenges become more manageable. Planning ahead for social events, finding carnivore-friendly restaurants, and developing strategies to handle cravings can help maintain your dietary goals.

The true reward of appreciating your carnivorous experience lies in the vision of a healthier future. By prioritizing your health and making informed dietary choices, you are investing in your long-term well-being. The reduction in chronic disease risk, improved metabolic health, and enhanced mental clarity are just a few of the benefits that pave the way for a vibrant, fulfilling life.

The journey doesn't end once you've adopted the carnivorous diet; it's an ongoing process of learning and adaptation. Staying informed about new research, listening to your body's responses, and making necessary adjustments ensures that your diet remains aligned with your health goals. This proactive approach fosters a deeper appreciation for your dietary choices and keeps you motivated to pursue optimal health.

Every milestone on your carnivorous journey is worth celebrating. Whether it's reaching a weight loss goal, experiencing relief from chronic symptoms, or simply feeling more energized, these successes are testaments to the effectiveness of the diet. Take time to acknowledge and celebrate these achievements, as they reinforce the positive impact of your carnivorous lifestyle.

Appreciating your carnivorous experience is about more than just adhering to a diet; it's about embracing a path to better health and well-being. By focusing on the transformative benefits, simplifying your nutritional approach, and engaging with a supportive community, you can fully enjoy and sustain your carnivorous lifestyle. With a hopeful outlook towards a healthier future, each step on this journey becomes a rewarding and empowering experience.

As you continue to navigate this unique dietary path, remember that your commitment to health is the greatest investment you can make for yourself.